The Little Book Of Acid

Cam Cloud

Ronin Publishing
Berkeley, CA

www.roninpub.com

The Little Book Of Acid

Cam Cloud

THE LITTLE BOOK OF ACID
ISBN: 0-914171-887
Copyright © 1999 by Ronin Publishing, Inc.

Published by RONIN PUBLISHING, INC.
PO Box 522
Berkeley, CA 94701
www.roninpub.com

Printed by Data Reproductions
Distributed by Publishers Group West

Project Editor: Dan Joy
Technical Editors: KT Carson and Christopher Delay
Cover Design: Judy July, Generic Type

First printing 1999
9 8 7 6 5 4 3 2 1

Notice To Readers

Manufacture, possession, use, and distribution of LSD are all serious crimes under Federal drug laws. It is illegal to possess, use, extract, or distribute lysergic acid amides—LSD's natural cousins from the plant world.

Solvents used to make extracts documented in this book are hazardous. Do not attempt these procedures. Not only can you land in jail, you can cause an explosion and inhale toxic fumes.

Psychedelic exploration presents its own inherent dangers. Psychedelic trips may not always be pleasant experiences. Lysergic acid amides and their plant sources can have unpleasant side effects and involve serious risks for pregnant women. Furthermore, tripping can change the way people think and how they choose to live, thereby challenging present lifestyle and personal status quo.

This material is presented as historical novelty and archive of certain underground culture and alchemical practices. The purpose of this book is not to advocate tripping, but to describe it for those who have a need to know or who are merely curious.

Ours is a free society and we are allowed to read about and discuss—even fantasize about—illicit matters. However, carrying out procedures documented in this book is risky to your health and to your freedom—and just plain stupid. The author and publisher urge readers to be smart and not to run a foul of the law. The author and publisher make no warranties of any kind, including accuracy, with respect to the information in this book and assume no responsibility for Readers who disregard this notice.

Table Of Contents

Introduction 1

1. What Is Acid? 3

2. The Trip 9

3. Afterglow 15

4. Bummers 21

5. Acid Underground 27

6. Blotter Acid 31

7. Barrels, Dots & Cubes 35

8. Acid Lingo 41

9. Psychedelic Vines 45

10. Tripping On Seeds 51

11. Cultivation 55

12. Preparation And Use 59

13. Psychedelic Seed Extracts . 65

14. How Extracts Are Made ... 71

15. Acid, Seeds, And The Law. 77

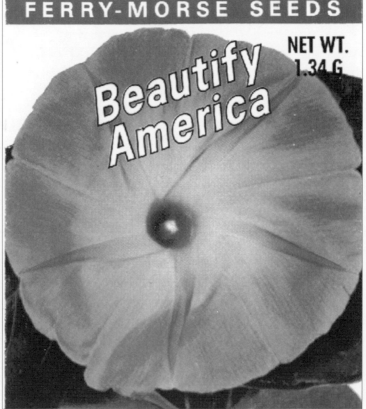

39¢

MORNING GLORY
HEAVENLY BLUE

FERRY-MORSE SEEDS

Beautify America

NET WT.
1.34 G

Seed contained herein is for planting purposes only

Introduction

 LSD-25, widely known simply as *acid* is one of the most potent substances ever discovered by humankind. It takes only a few millionths of a gram—a literally microscopic amount—for a trip. Acid's effects on the mind are so remarkable that this chemical has generated decades of excitement as well as social and political conflict. Entire subcultures, social movements, and forms of art and music have arisen from its use. A huge body of laws and massive law enforcement efforts have been created to control the manufacture, distribution, and consumption of this substance. Acid is probably the most controversial drug of all time.

Other books about psychedelics are lengthy, dense, and hard to comprehend, tending to reflect only the perspective of one particular scientific or scholarly discipline, like chemistry, psychology, or history. Many are autobiographical, detailing only one person's acid experiences. Readers interested in the subject for whatever reason must wade through a vast expanse of difficult material to assemble a clear picture of basic issues concerned with acid.

The Little Book of Acid is clear, simple and straightforward. It describes essential aspects of acid, discusses how people use and think about it. It talks about what tripping feels like, how people go about tripping, and how they encourage good trips and handle bad ones. It also explains different ways that acid is packaged, sold, distributed and consumed.

The Little Book of Acid focuses on the natural plant sources of LSD-like chemicals, describing the psychedelic properties and how they were discovered. It discusses how the plants themselves, as well as organic extractions made from them, are cultivated and used to trip.

The Little Book of Acid describes on the thriving present-day acid underground—the colorful, creative, vibrant subculture that has grown up around acid and the knowledge, commerce, and practices that it has spawned.

A great deal of important information about tripping has been discovered within the acid underground. Much of this insight, as well as information about the acid underground itself, is rarely published—despite the fact that "underground" is where almost all the acid action has taken place since it was declared illegal many years ago. *The Little Book Of Acid* fills this gap—while taking care to distinguish between reality and the often erroneous folklore and mythology that circulates in underground circles along with solid, hard-earned trip wisdom.

Cam Cloud

1

What Is Acid?

 Known to chemists as "lysergic acid diethy-
lamide-25," acid is a "semi-synthetic"
chemical compound—meaning it is part
natural and part man-made. In other words, acid is a
laboratory modification of a naturally-occurring
substance. It is created by combining a chemical
called "diethylamine" with lysergic acids, substances that are found naturally in certain molds and
plants.

Acid belongs to a family of chemicals called
"tryptamines," named for the presence in the mol-
ecule of an ammonia-like configuration called an
"amine group." Tryptamines of
various kinds are common in
nature, and several tryptamines
occur naturally in the human
brain. Many psychedelic drugs
in addition to LSD such as DMT
and psilocybin—are also
tryptamines.

**Lysergic Acid
Diethylcomide-25**

Your Brain On Acid

Like other psychoactive drugs,
acid works by interacting with

the brain. Only a tiny fraction, however, of the acid that a person ingests—which is a very minute quantity to begin with—actually finds its way into the brain. This fact underscores just how incredibly potent acid really is.

Once in the brain, acid is believed to work primarily upon networks of brain cells that interact closely with serotonin, the most widely known of all brain chemicals. Serotonin performs a vast array of physiological functions in the body in addition to playing a key role in the regulation of mood, sensation, and consciousness. Many antidepressant drugs, including the popular Prozac®, also act on the brain's serotonin systems. Aside from its poorly understood relationship to serotonin, hardly anything is known about how acid generates its effects.

Your Body On Acid

For a drug of such amazing potency, acid has remarkably little effect on the human body. Its impact on physiological processes is exceedingly minor. Pulse, blood pressure, and body temperature go up slightly, production of saliva increases, the pupils of the eyes usually dilate somewhat—and that's about it.

Acid causes no known harm to human cells, tissues, or organs, and no lethal dosage level of the drug has ever been established. Acid does not show up on drug tests. In fact, ninety percent of any dose of acid disappears from the body *before* its peak effects are felt! Acid's extraordinary power, then, bypasses the human body to concentrate almost wholly on the human mind.

What is "Psychedelic"?

The term "psychedelic" was coined in the 1950s in correspondence between visionary novelist Aldous Huxley and psychiatrist Humphrey Osmond. It comes from two Greek roots: the word *psyche*, which means "mind" or "soul," and *deloun*, which means "to make manifest" or "to reveal." A "psychedelic," therefore, is a substance that reveals the nature of the mind or soul.

Writer Laura Huxley, wife of Aldus Huxley and a therapist, described psychedelics as "stimulators of ideas and feelings." The effects of classical psychedelics, which include LSD, mescaline, DMT, and psilocybin, are characterized by alterations of sensory perception and intensification of both external sensory phenomena and internal feelings and thoughts. Psychedelics are especially known for generating spiritual, mystical, and visionary experiences.

The Discovery of Acid

Acid was first synthesized in 1938 by chemist Albert Hofmann of the Sandoz pharmaceutical company in Switzerland. It was not until 1943, however, that Hofmann became the first person ever to experience the remarkable drug, which would probably have remained unknown to this day but for the coincidential mix of whim and accident that made its discovery possible.

Hofmann synthesized the drug originally as part of a series of derivatives of a grain mold—actually a tiny mushroom—called ergot. These substances were being investigated for possible use in obstetrics as well as other medical applications. When uninter-

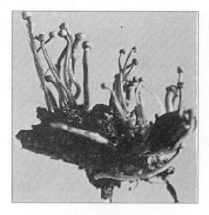

Sclerotium of ergot of rye enlarged enormously

esting results were produced by animal tests with LSD-25—the twenty-fifth in this series of compounds to be created—research was abandoned, and Hofman forgot about it.

Five years later, however, Hofmann was inexplicably driven by what he called a "peculiar presentiment"—in other words, a feeling of precognition—to make LSD-25 again.

As a precise professional chemist, Hofmann always followed strict protocols and rigorous precautions. His exacting work habits make it surprising that, when he made LSD-25 for the second time, he somehow managed get some of it into his system, later he speculated that it was probably absorbed through the skin of his fingers.

Hofmann began to experience strange changes in consciousness that made it impossible for him to continue working. Concerned for his safety, he had his assistant accompany him on his bicycle ride home, where he was destined to experience the world's first acid trip.

Hofmann didn't know what had caused this mysterious episode, but careful reasoning suggested to him that it had been the LSD-25. He confirmed this hypothesis the next week by intentionally ingesting a very small amount of the substance that sent him off on a profound psychedelic journey. Hofmann reported his results to his superiors, and Sandoz soon began marketing the intriguing but mystifying compound under the trade name "Delysid," making it available to researchers only.

Acid Travels Around the World

Since Hofmann's fateful first trip, acid has been the subject of volumes of clinical research and more than a decade of top-secret, top-priority military experiments. It has been the object of widespread fear, confusion, panic, hysteria, and media sensationalism. It was central to the youth rebellions of the 1960s— one of the century's most tumultuous cultural upheavals—when it was championed with evangelistic fervor and demonized with equal zeal. Legions were convinced that it could save the world, while equal numbers insisted that it could destroy an entire generation of youth.

A key figure in the popularization of acid was psychologist Timothy Leary. Along with other members of Harvard University's psychology department, Leary conducted a series of explosively controversial research programs with acid and other psychedelics that ultimately resulted in his dismissal from Harvard amidst enormous publicity. For the next several years, Leary and his group kept up their research without academic auspices, and massive media attention followed Leary and his activities for the rest of his life.

The press described Leary as a proselytizer and "acid guru," creating an image far too exaggerated to reflect the truth. Leary was actually an anti-authoritarian who was wary of "gurus" on principle and didn't like having submissive fans. His attitude about tripping was considerably more cautionary than most portrayals suggest, and became even more reserved as the years went by. In fact—at least on an individual basis—Leary often advised people *against* using acid and other drugs, emphasizing the high level of responsibility required.

From hundreds of his own trips and thousands that he guided, supervised, or witnessed, Leary accumulated an extraordinary understanding of tripping—including important cautionary principles that he articulated with exceptional clarity. For this reason, Leary's acid wisdom is frequently drawn upon in this book.

Acid Becomes a Crime

In 1967—just as acid was becoming a religious sacrament for scores of alternative churches and thousands of sincere spiritual seekers—the controversial psychedelic was banned in the United States. Manufacture, distribution, and use of LSD soon became crimes of utmost seriousness in many other nations of the world as well.

Widespread legal restrictions notwithstanding, acid has been a key catalyst in the birth and development of the dozens of "new paradigms"—or innovative schools of thought—that have proliferated in science, psychology, politics, and spirituality with the approach new millennium. And the availability and popularity of the drug are, by all indications, surging upward once again.

2

The Trip

The experience of an acid trip can go in a virtually infinite number of directions. No two acid trips are the same, even for experienced trippers. Acid alters perception, awakens memories, heightens emotion, and changes thinking patterns. Acid often stimulates creativity, and can open the door to spiritual experiences.

Heightening of Senses

Acid amplifies all of the senses to create a sensory experience of extraordinary intensity, richness, subtlety, and depth. An endlessly fascinating world of new detail opens to the eye. Previously overlooked facets of light, shading, and texture become apparent. Everything seems to be in motion: trees breathe, walls ripple, and normally dull surfaces sparkle and vibrate.

Often the environment appears to arrange itself into a perfectly harmonious composition like a great work of art. Previously unheard oscillations, reverberations, and overtones open up new dimensions in sound. Music becomes heavenly, art becomes overwhelmingly beautiful, and landscapes become breathtaking. Timothy Leary once called this experi-

ence a "Niagara of sensory input" after the huge
cascading waterfall in upstate New York.

Visuals

Trippers use the word "visuals" to refer to the
visual impressions and images that acid can generate. There are various kinds of visuals.

Strikingly detailed, luminescent shapes, images,
and panoramas ranging from abstract geometric
forms to populous landscapes often appear before
the closed eyes of a person under the influence of a
strong dose of acid. These constantly changing
images, which can be transcendentally beautiful or
utterly horrifying, are called "eidetic imagery" by
scientists and "closed-eye visuals" by many trippers.

Another common-acid generated visual experience—which, unlike eidetic imagery, occurs when
the eyes are open—involves highly ordered, complex, often geometrical forms and shapes that appear on the surfaces of objects, especially large blank
expanses like white walls. These repetitive, tapestry-
like patterns move, grow, ripple, and swirl, and can
decorate the tripper's visual world like wallpaper.
Trippers call them simply "patterns"—or sometimes
"paisleys," after a shape that commonly appears in
these patterns.

Another frequent visual phenomenon is known
as "trails." These are sequences of repeating multiple
after-images left behind by an object moving across
the visual field, like the ripples created by something
moving across the surface of a pond. This visual
effect has become almost synonymous with tripping
itself; some trippers wish each other good acid trips
with the phrase, "Happy Trails!"

Senses Overlap

Under the influence of acid, the different senses
often seem to cross over into one another. For instance, a color may emit a sound, a sound may have
a color, or odors may have color and sound. This
effect is called *synesthesia*. In Timothy Leary's words,
"when your nervous system is turned on with LSD,
and all the wires are flashing, the senses begin to
overlap and merge. You not only hear but see the
music emerging from the speaker system—like

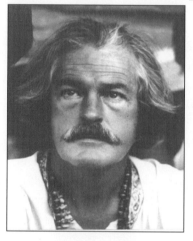

dancing particles, like
squirming curls of
toothpaste. You actually
see the sound in multi-
layered patterns while
you're hearing it."

Time Slows Down

The passage of time
seems to slow down
tremendously when
under the influence of
acid. A few minutes
may seem like hours; a

Timothy Leary

few hours may seem like days. This effect is known
as "time dilation." At the peak of a very powerful
trip it may seem as if time has come to a complete
stop, plunging the tripper into a timeless, eternal
realm.

Thinking Is Freed Up

Acid frees the tripper's thinking from its habitual
patterns, opening the mind to a flood of often aston-
ishing new ideas and images. Acid accelerates the

mental process that psychologists call "free association," in which one thought leads to another in a
series of novel links. Normal linear step-by-step
thinking, closely connected to words, gives way to
the pattern-oriented, intuitive, imagistic kind of
thinking associated with the activity of the right lobe
of the brain. Sometimes under a strong dose of acid
the thinking process goes beyond words entirely, a
rare phenomenon that occurs almost exclusively in
altered states of awareness.

Expanded Sense of Self

Acid trips are characterized by a loosening of the
sense of separation between the internal self and the
external world. This quality often leads to a sense of
oneness with other people and the world. Feelings
of telepathic contact with others and with animals
are common. Such experiences often create bonding
between people who trip together, who may feel as
if they have seen deeply into one another's souls.

Some people even experience communication
with plants and trees when they trip. At higher
dosages there may be a sensation of merging with
the universe, of becoming mystically "one with
everything."

Psychological Breakthroughs

Acid is associated with heightened intensity of
emotion. Both positive and negative emotions are
amplified and can become exquisitely powerful.

Acid trips also often bring into consciousness
memories that have been lost or buried. These
memories can be experienced quite vividly, as if they
were being re-lived.

Psychotherapy is often geared towards revealing and putting the client in touch with his or her feelings. Many forms of therapy also focus on bringing lost memories of traumatic early events into the forefront of the client's awareness. Because acid both amplifies emotion and awakens lost memory, there was once a great deal of enthusiasm among therapists and psychiatrists regarding acid's potential to deepen and accelerate psychotherapy. Before acid was declared illegal, more than 40,000 people received it in conjunction with psychotherapy.

Enhanced Creativity

Acid experiences are widely connected to breakthroughs in creativity and problem-solving. Many trippers, for instance, have reported that solutions to previously insoluble problems have occurred to them during acid trips. Several writers have said that acid has helped them break free of writer's block.

Before LSD was made illegal, at least nine major scientific studies were conducted exploring the drug's stimulating impact on creativity. Frank Barron, the psychologist who "turned on" Timothy Leary, specialized in the study of psychedelics and creativity, as did the world-renowned psychiatrist Oscar Janiger. Surveys on the subject suggest that acid stimulates creativity only among those already concerned with creativity. No artist in any survey conducted on the issue ever reported that acid *diminished* his or her creativity.

Spiritual Awakenings

People who take acid often report experiences that they describe as powerful spiritual awakenings. Acid trips of this kind have made mystics, religious converts, and spiritual practitioners out of many trippers. The spiritual potential of LSD was an important factor behind the tripping explosion of the 1960s, and it has continued to fuel underground acid experimentation ever since.

Psychedelics have played a role in spirituality and religion for thousands of years. Organic psychedelics such as psilocybin mushrooms and ayahuasca have been used in initiations, healing practices, and religious ceremonies by tribal peoples since before the dawn of history. Today, the Native American Church still uses the psychedelic peyote cactus in its rituals, with legal protection from the United States Government on the grounds of religious freedom. The connection between psychedelics and spiritual experience has led ethnobotanical researcher Jonathan Ott to popularize the term "entheogen" to refer to substances that have the capacity to generate inner experiences of God, gods, or divinity.

3

Afterglow

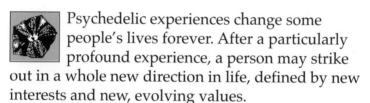Psychedelic experiences change some people's lives forever. After a particularly profound experience, a person may strike out in a whole new direction in life, defined by new interests and new, evolving values.

Whether or not a trip triggers this kind of deep transformation, it is likely to effect how a person thinks and feels for days, weeks, or months afterwards—just like any other significant experience. A person who has had a spiritual experience on acid, for instance, may continue to have spontaneous spiritual feelings for a while. A person who has had a creative breakthrough usually continues to be more creative, especially so in the days following the trip. When a trip has been disturbing or frightening, feelings of this kind may persist like a bad "aftertaste."

Pure acid doesn't cause any known physiological stress or damage and therefore doesn't cause a "hangover" like so many other recreational drugs, from alcohol to ecstasy. Many people, however, are tired out the day after a trip just as they might be after a hike or outing.

Stimulation

Although the experience of tripping and acid's physiological route of action are both very different from those of typical "uppers," acid is nonetheless a stimulant which increases the level of activity in the nervous system. Lacking the harsh edge and crashing "come-downs" associated with stronger stimulants like speed or coke, acid's mild stimulant effect often lingers for a while after the psychedelic effects have dissipated. For this reason, many people have trouble sleeping for several hours after a trip is over, even though they may feel tired out.

Many trippers just let this stimulation run its course, remaining awake but in a restful situation, enjoying the reverberations of their experience and not trying to sleep until their bodies are naturally ready to do so. Others may feel a more insistent need to sleep, to "turn off" after "turning on." They may use over-the-counter sleeping aids or mild doses of prescription tranquilizers like Valium® to help them get to sleep. Other trippers sometimes find that antihistamines are all that's needed to effectively promote sleep, while some prefer to drink a little alcohol to "smooth the jitters." None of these drugs has dangerous interactions with LSD, but mixing alcohol with tranquilizers is very risky.

Afterglow

For many people, the day after an acid trip can be an especially enjoyable day, particularly if the trip was a very good one. They may enjoy a lingering, pleasurable heightening of the senses and pleasant echoes of the psychedelic spaces that they have traversed, an "afterglow" in which the world appears fresh, bright, and new.

In *LSD: My Problem Child*, Albert Hofmann, the Swiss chemist who discovered LSD, describes the afterglow he experienced after one of his first trips. After getting some sleep, he awakened "refreshed, with a clear head, though still somewhat tired physically.

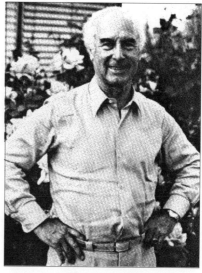

Albert Hofmann

A sensation of well-being and renewed life flowed through me. Breakfast tasted delicious and gave me extraordinary pleasure. When I later walked out into the garden, in which the sun shone now after a spring rain, everything glistened and sparkled in a fresh light. The world was as if newly created. All my senses vibrated in a condition of highest sensitivity, which persisted for the entire day."

Recovery

Many trippers take the day after an acid trip off, planning in advance so that they will be free from any major responsibilities. This practice allows them to recover from insomnia or fatigue that may have resulted from the trip. It also creates an opportunity to meditate upon the meaning and implications of their psychedelic adventure, to absorb and integrate the experience to some degree before moving back into the hustle and bustle of daily life. If the trip was a difficult one, taking the next day off provides time to work on shaking off leftover negative feelings, while if the trip was a good one, it creates an opportunity to bask in the afterglow.

Are Flashbacks Real?

It's widely believed—especially among people who have never taken acid—that a person who has had even just one trip can experience a disruptive mental phenomenon called "flashbacks" for months or even years afterwards. The myth of the flashback was widely promoted by the media and government as one of the severe dangers of LSD.

According to descriptions of flashbacks that have circulated in anti-LSD propaganda and popular folklore, the person is suddenly and without warning plunged into a full-on psychedelic state even though no acid has been taken. The person can't terminate the flashback and has no influence over how long it lasts. A flashback, therefore, amounts to complete loss of control of one's consciousness, an especially serious hazard if one is alone, in a public place, or driving a car.

People who have taken acid as well as scientists and psychologists and who have studied the phenomenon of LSD use report that flashbacks of this kind are a myth. Some people who use acid, however, note an increased flexibility of consciousness, consisting of easier access to altered states and heightened awareness which become more available both spontaneously and through applied effort. Similar effects have been reported by people who practice meditation and other means of promoting altered states.

Certain aspects of psychedelic consciousness, it seems, can be learned like any other skill. These phenomena are not nearly as dramatic or overwhelming as the "flashback" of pop culture mythology, but they probably explain how this myth originated.

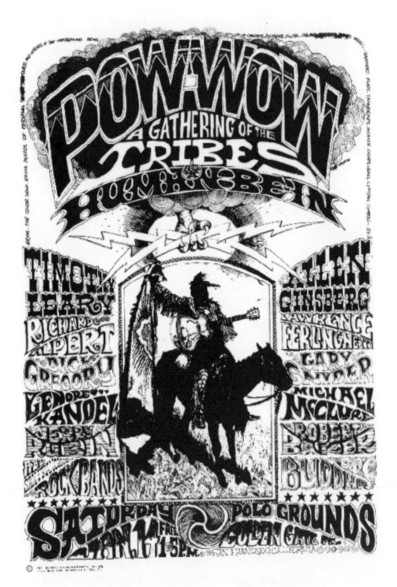

Acid art poster for the Be-In held in San Francisco's
Golden Gate Park January 14, 1967.

4

Bummers

 Acid can magnify negative, unpleasant perceptions and feelings just as it magnifies positive, enjoyable ones. Therefore, while acid trips can be ecstatically pleasurable, they can also be extremely unpleasant—even nightmarish. Trippers call unpleasant acid experiences "bummers" or "bad trips." It can take days or even weeks to completely shake off the negative mental and emotional residue that sometimes lingers in the wake of a particularly intense bummer. Bad trips have compelled some trippers to forswear acid altogether.

Negative Experiences

During bad trips, people can experience profound confusion, deep despair, intense fear, and feelings of horror. The time-expanding effects of acid can make these sensations seem to last for excruciatingly long periods of time. The tripper may lose touch with the fact that these are *temporary* effects related to the ingestion of a drug. This confusion can compound the suffering already taking place with a fear that it will go on forever.

Overwhelmed trippers may, in fact, completely forget that they are tripping. Such disconnection with reality presents the danger of drifting off into a private, subjective world—getting lost in an interior landscape of darkness, foreboding, and delusion that the tripper mistakes for the objective or "real" external world.

How Bummers Are Minimized

The good news is that bad trips—like all trips—inevitably come to an end. Furthermore, bad trips are prevented—or at least minimized—by thoughtful attention to the key factors that influence the nature and course of trips. These factors are easily understood, and are used as guiding principles when planning and preparing for trips. This practice balances the scales in favor of enjoyable, rewarding psychedelic experiences.

What Influences A Trip?

The three crucial influences that shape people's experiences with psychoactive substances are called "dosage, set, and setting." "Dosage" refers to the amount of the drug that is taken. "Set" refers to the state of mind of the person who takes the drug. "Setting" refers to the environment in which the drug experience occurs.

Dosage

Crisis-level bummers are less likely to happen on low doses of acid—100 mikes or less—than on high doses of 150 mikes or more. A tripper on a low dose is less likely to become so overwhelmed by negative sensations that he or she loses behavioral discretion or touch with reality. A tripper on a low dose is more in control of mental processes and therefore more capable of thinking or talking his or her way out of a negative state of mind. People on low doses are also usually more competent to make and execute decisions about changes of setting that might favorably alter the nature of the trip.

Furthermore, a person bumming out on a low dose is easier for others to communicate with than a person bumming out on a high dose, who may find verbal communication unusually challenging. Low doses thus present greater opportunity for companions to help change the course of the trip by talking with the tripper.

Set

People who are in a good mood at the time of a trip—relatively free from stress and enjoying life in general—are likely to have good trips. On the other hand, disturbing or emotionally disruptive personal issues—from financial stress to marital tension or recent loss—are likely to cause bummers. For this reason, adept trippers make a practice of evaluating their present emotional and mental state when deciding to trip. They look at current life stresses and preoccupations to determine if these influences are of sufficient magnitude to turn a psychedelic experience sour. This pre-trip assessment helps prevent bummers.

Expectations, preconceptions, and beliefs about acid and tripping in general are also an influential aspect of set. People with fearful or negative attitudes towards acid are more likely to have bad trips.

Setting

The environment in which a person trips has such a profound impact on the nature of the experience that inappropriate settings may be the foremost cause of bad trips. Tripping at school or on the job—settings frequently chosen by inexperienced youth, according to a study on LSD use conducted in the early 1990s—invites problems because of the pressures and restrictions inherent in such environments.

Choice of setting is an individual matter. A setting that feels safe and comfortable for one person may provoke anxiety in another. Even seemingly low-key, relaxed situations can be very stimulating to a tripping person. Crowded public places can be utterly overwhelming under the influence of acid, even to those who normally have no anxiety about such situations. While experienced trippers may enjoy doing acid at rock concerts, raves, or fairs, many still in the process of getting their psychedelic "sea-legs" have discovered the benefits of tripping only in especially serene environments until they are accustomed to the sensory amplification that acid generates. To avoid undesirable interruptions that can disrupt a good trip, many people disconnect the doorbell and turn off the phone for the duration of a trip.

Influences of Other People

A crucial aspect of setting is the other people present when a person takes a trip. While interpersonal interaction can be an exquisitely rewarding dimension of tripping, it is also a source of bummers.

Companions may result in problems for the tripper in a number of ways. Disagreements may arise as to how time during the trip is to be spent. Previously unexamined interpersonal issues and conflicts may come to the fore and dominate the trip. The heightened emotional and sensory awareness engendered by LSD may cause facets of another person's behavior or personality that are normally inconsequential to become excruciatingly exaggerated. Another's reserved manner, for instance, may be experienced by the tripper as emotional abandonment. And the dissolution of interpersonal boundaries that occurs with acid can cause another person's discomfort, anxiety, or neurosis to be felt as intensely as if it were the tripper's own.

Because of these factors, discriminating trippers choose as companions only people that they are very comfortable with, know well, and are willing to get to know better.

Handling Bummers

No matter what precautions are taken with regard to dosage, set, and setting, bummers still happen. Through years of trial and error, many trippers have developed skill at handling the bad trips of others.

People looking after someone who is having a bad trip remove disturbing influences—sources of unpleasant noise and interruption—and get the person to a safe, comforting environment in which stimulation is reduced. All the while, they reassure the tripper in a soothing manner. If the tripper fears that he or she is going crazy, they remind him or her that the experience is being caused by a drug and will be over with in a few hours. If tripper is disturbed by odd bodily sensations, they reassure him or her that the body is actually functioning normally. Particularly important is refocusing the person's attention onto positive and beautiful elements of the environment like flowers, trees, and works of art.

Anxiety can be reduced with tranquilizers like Valium®, but most people experienced in handling bummers agree that it's not usually worth it to take the tripper to a clinic or hospital emergency room in order to obtain such medication. These settings—which are full of strangers, bright lights, tension, and noise—tend to make bad trips even worse.

People experienced with acid recommend calm, supportive conversation as the best method for reducing panic. Too much talking or lengthy intellectual digressions, however, may be overwhelming or difficult for the tripper to follow. Experienced companions speak straightforwardly, using simple, soothing words.

5

Acid Underground

 Acid became illegal in 1967. Since then, a worldwide underground economy centered around the manufacture and distribution of acid has evolved. This network has its own corporation-like organizations and structures, the upper echelons of which have managed to evade drug enforcement authorities for years. The San Francisco Bay Area is a major global center of LSD production and distribution.

The Drug Enforcement Administration (DEA) constantly tracks the acid underground. In fact, much of the information in this chapter comes from the DEA.

Idealism

One factor that sharply distinguishes the acid underground from most other illicit enterprises is its idealistic character. Many participants in the underground are motivated as much by their belief in acid's spiritual benefits as by the desire to make money. If money were their sole motive, most of these people would have found a less risky way to make it.

In this regard, the acid underground retains much of the missionary fervor that fueled multitudes of youth during the 1960s LSD explosion. Many participants in today's acid underground view themselves as keeping alive the flame of this "psychedelic revolution."

Drug enforcement authorities acknowledge the important role this idealistic vision has played in shaping and maintaining the acid underground that they have been trying to dismantle for decades. One DEA report states, "LSD trafficking has assumed an ideological or crusading aspect . . . belief in the beneficent properties of LSD has been, over the years, as strong a motivating factor in the production and distribution of the drug as the profits to be made from its sale."

Evolution of the Underground

Ergotamine tartrate, a substance extracted from a species of rye mold called ergot, is the primary

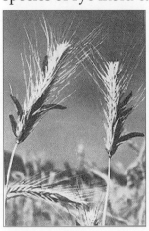

Rye

starting material used in the production of LSD. Different phases in the development of the acid underground have been marked by different means of procuring ergotamine tartrate. During the early days of the underground, acid was supplied by various small groups that got limited quantities of ergotamine tartrate from the legitimate commercial chemical-supply market.

A group that obtained large amounts of ergotamine tartrate from Mexico and Costa Rica became the main source of underground acid for the entire United States at the end of the 1960s. Law enforcement shut down this group in the early 1970s. Then another organization became the principal source of acid. This group bought ergotamine tartrate from legitimate domestic suppliers through the use of front companies. Drug enforcement authorities managed to neutralize this organization as well, and believed that they had wiped out large-scale production and distribution of LSD in the United States—a conviction supported by a dramatic drop in the amount of illicit acid seized by drug enforcement agents.

This situation, however, didn't last long. By 1976, another organization, centered in the San Francisco Bay Area, assumed the primary role in the production and distribution of acid. According to the DEA, this organization managed virtually the entire acid market by controlling the importation of illicit ergotamine tartrate and franchising acid production rights. It obtained its ergotamine tartrate from smugglers supplied by European underground organizations that in turn acquired it from legitimate European chemical firms. According to the DEA, no significant diversions of ergotamine tartrate from legitimate domestic sources has taken place since this group's rise to prominence.

The San Francisco group shipped liquid acid to areas in the United States where demand was greatest and to primarily English-speaking overseas locations. The liquid was applied to blotter paper by operations located at these destinations.

Acid Distribution

Acid is readily available in retail quantities in every state of the United States. Northern California is the source of supply for most LSD available in the nation. At the wholesale production and trafficking level, LSD is controlled tightly by California-based groups that have operated with relative impunity for decades.

Distributors often pay for supply by Western Union wire or with postal money orders. Upon receipt of payment, acid is shipped to the distributor. At the retail level, acid is sold almost exclusively on a cash-and-carry basis. Money laundering is not generally conducted on a sophisticated level in the acid underground except by international traffickers.

Federal Express and other overnight delivery services are used to transport large amounts of acid from the San Francisco Bay Area to locations throughout the United States. Acid is frequently concealed in greeting cards, cassette tapes, or articles of clothing mailed to a post office box which is usually listed under a fictitious name. Normally, no return address appears on the package or envelope.

Retail-level acid distribution networks in the United States are generally comprised of individuals who have known each other through long association and common interests. The cohesiveness of these communities facilitates not only hand-to-hand sales but a proliferation of mail order business.

6
Blotter Acid

 Blotter acid is the most common form in which acid is packaged, sold, and consumed today. Blotter acid is paper which has been soaked in a liquid solution of LSD. The liquid evaporates off, leaving the paper impregnated with acid. The paper is perforated to create row upon row of little squares—usually about a quarter of an inch square—each of which holds one hit of acid that is usually around 65 mikes in strength.

Designs

Some sheets of blotter acid are blank, but most have been printed with designs. Sometimes the design takes up the entire sheet, so that only a small piece of the design is visible on a single hit—something like a jigsaw puzzle. Most sheets, however, are printed in such a way that a complete tiny design appears on each piece or hit. Sometimes several such designs appear on a single sheet.

Blotter acid has sported a variety of creative, fanciful images. Several varieties of widely distributed blotter acid have featured cartoon characters such as Donald Duck, Goofy, and Mickey Mouse in his incarnation as the wand-wielding wizard from

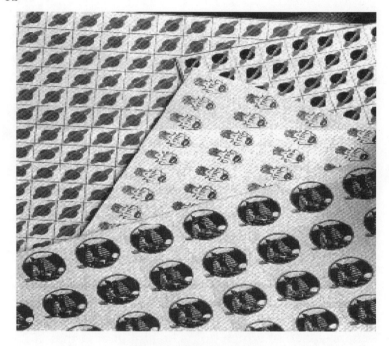

Sheets of blotter acid

the movie *Fantasia*. This use of cartoon images pro-
voked alarm among parents and authorities that
acid was being purposefully packaged in such a way
as to appeal to children—a charge that those in the
acid underground considered absurd.

Symbols of mystical, spiritual, or occult significance, such as alchemical wheels, the Hindu el-
ephant-deity Ganesh, eye-in-the-pyramid triangles,
and lotus flowers are also frequently used. Dragons
in a range of colors, robots, suns with smiling faces,
Celtic latticeworks, family crests, and rainbow
spectra have appeared on acid blotter paper. One
series of blotter prints featured tiny portraits of
luminaries from LSD history including Timothy
Leary and Albert Hofmann.

Underground acid manufacturers often put a great deal of thought, effort, and care into this artistic dimension of their work. Designs used on blotter art over the years have been so striking, colorful, and distinctive—and, needless to say, psychedelic in style—that blotter art has become an art form unto itself. Entire gallery art shows have used it as a theme.

Making Blotter Acid

After the sheets of paper have been printed and perforated, liquid LSD is applied to them—a process called "laying sheets"—and they are left to dry. The facilities for performing this operation are easily set up, used, broken down, and transported. People operating sheet-laying facilities, which the DEA calls "conversion laboratories," move the operation around to keep a step ahead of the law, setting up shop in a series of different apartments, motel rooms, and recreational vehicles.

Sheets are impregnated with acid by dipping them into a shallow pan containing LSD crystal dissolved in a solvent such as methanol or ethanol. Water is not used because it takes longer to evaporate, necessitating a greater time period during which the drying sheets are exposed to light, heat, or other factors that cause degradation of LSD into inactive chemicals.

LSD is so potent that quantities having a very strong psychedelic effect can be absorbed through the skin or by breathing microscopic airborne particles. People laying sheets often wear rubber gloves, breathing masks, and even goggles to prevent accidental ingestion. Even with such precautions, however, they often still get high during the process.

Quantities

Blotter acid is sold in various units. Single hits or small clusters of them are sold on the retail level to individual trippers. A "sheet" is one hundred hits on a ten-by-ten-hit piece of paper, a unit often sold on the retail level. A larger piece of paper consisting of ten unseparated sheets—a thousand hits, known as a "page"—is a unit commonly sold wholesale. Ten pages—ten thousand hits—constitute a "book," which is a common wholesale unit.

Cost

The per-hit cost of acid drops sharply as the quantity purchased increases. The price of acid over the last several decades has been subject to very little inflation as compared to prices for marijuana and other underground drugs, which have skyrocketed. The stability in the cost of acid is probably connected to the idealistic character of the LSD underground, reflecting a desire to give customers a good deal and keep the mystical psychedelic available to large numbers of people.

The average retail price of acid is $5 per hit, while lots of a thousand are often sold for less than a dollar per hit. These low prices make acid a bargain compared to other recreational drugs, especially considering the duration of its effects. A hit of Ecstasy, for example, lasts a maximum of six hours, costing as much as $25, while six hours worth of cocaine can run into the hundreds of dollars. By comparison, trippers get eight to twelve hours of psychedelic reverie for only $5—even less than the cost of a movie!

7

Barrels, Dots & Cubes

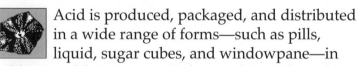 Acid is produced, packaged, and distributed in a wide range of forms—such as pills, liquid, sugar cubes, and windowpane—in addition to blotter paper. Before acid is packaged in any of these forms, however, it is produced as a crystal, the end-product created when LSD is synthesized in a chemical laboratory.

Crystal Acid

Crystalline acid appears only at the highest levels of underground distribution networks because of a variety of factors that make handling and distribution of this material unsafe and impractical. Foremost among these is the tremendous potency of unprocessed crystal LSD. An amount of crystal that is almost too small to be seen with the naked eye is nonetheless sufficient to produce a very strong trip. Such a speck of acid can easily become airborne and land on someone's skin or find its way into a breath of air, thereby getting absorbed into the body and causing an unexpected trip. In fact, crystal acid is so potent that people often seem to end up getting high merely from being around it. Another reason for packaging LSD into other forms is the suspicion aroused by crystalline powders. Furthermore, crystal acid is especially susceptible to decomposition by heat and light.

Crystal acid is usually transported and sold in plastic film canisters, small opaque plastic bottles, or other containers that provide protection from degradation. Crystal acid that has been subjected to oxidation—one of the main types of decomposition to which LSD is vulnerable—turns darker than its proper white or slightly off-white color. Crystal acid displaying this telltale sign of decomposition is generally considered unfit for sale.

Liquid Acid

Acid dissolved in liquid solutions is associated with mid-level distribution. Liquid acid is much easier to handle and transport than crystal. Because the acid becomes invisible in solution, liquid acid doesn't arouse suspicion as readily as crystal.

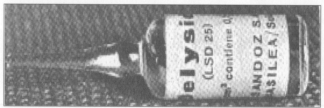

Ampule of legally manufactured liquid LSD

Much of the liquid acid produced is destined for conversion laboratories, where it will be applied to blotter paper or packaged in some other form.

Liquid acid is also sometimes used for human consumption. In this case, the acid has been dissolved in water instead of the toxic solvents in which acid destined for conversion to blotter paper is dissolved. It is usually diluted sufficiently as to require at least one drop to cause a trip, and is often packaged in a small bottle that has a dropper attached to the lid—just like herbal tinctures and homeopathic remedies sold in health food stores. The dropper assists in measuring out consistent doses.

Liquid acid is never made with tap water, which contains chemicals that rapidly degrade LSD into substances that have no psychoactive effects. Distilled water is necessary for making a stable solution.

Barrels

Acid was once commonly pressed into pills, a form in which it still occasionally appears today. Acid pills roughly the shape and size of aspirin tablets are called "barrels" because of their cylindrical shape. The famous "Orange Sunshine" acid of the late 1960s consisted of orange-colored barrels of this kind.

When acid is pressed into pills, it is mixed in with binders that make the pill solid and provide most of its bulk. Samples of barrels from all over the country were analyzed in the 1970s, revealing exactly the same composition of ingredients. This finding suggested to the authorities either that a single network was manufacturing all the pill-form acid in the country or that underground chemists were all using the same recipe.

Barrel acid declined in popularity for a number of reasons. The pill presses required to manufacture it are expensive, require skill to operate, need maintenance, can break down, and wear out with use. Pill presses are conspicuous when transported and require security to house and operate. The pills produced can break and crumble into powder under pressure or with the passage of time. Blotter thus turned out to be a much cheaper, more efficient, and safer way to package acid.

Microdots

Very tiny, often brightly-colored pills called "microdots" or "dots" still appear with some regularity in the underground acid market. The microdot form is possible because acid is so potent that these mini-pills, tiny though they are, are still big enough to hold an effective dose.

Certain very potent chemical cousins of mescaline are also packaged in microdot form. The resulting product is sometimes sold on the underground market as acid—or as mescaline, even though mescaline itself is not actually potent enough to package in microdots.

Sugar Cubes

Hits of liquid acid dropped onto sugar cubes made the legend of acid in the 1960s. Psychedelic art and psychedelic rock songs made reference to sugar cubes, which still sometimes appear today. Since sugar cubes crumble and melt easily, the acid is usually dropped onto the cube shortly before it is sold or consumed.

Windowpane

Sometimes acid is suspended in a solution that solidifies as a super-thin sheet of clear or translucent gelatin called "windowpane." The gelatin is often impregnated with brightly-colored dyes, and is sometimes allowed to harden in a mold which forms each individual hit to into a three-dimensional shape. In the early 1980s, a creative combination of these packaging techniques resulted in glittering iridescent sheets of purple or green windowpane acid, each hit of which was a tiny, sparkling, fully three-dimensional pyramid! This enchanting product represented one of the greatest heights of artistry ever achieved in drug packaging.

Windowpane is associated with potent doses of pure LSD. Hits of windowpane dissolve in the mouth like candy. The popularity of windowpane peaked in the 1970s, its prevalence declining sharply thereafter. Windowpane is considered a true connoisseur's rarity on today's underground acid market.

Cost, Potency, and Purity

The cost of liquid, barrels, microdots, windowpane, or sugar cubes is usually about the same as that of blotter acid. These varieties, however, are less common than in the 1960s and early 1970s before blotter acid rose to prominence.

According to the DEA, the potency of a hit of acid—whatever its form—is usually in the range of 20 to 80 mikes. This is a relatively mild dose compared to the 100- to 200-mike doses common in the 1960s.

Chemical analyses of samples seized by government authorities over the years show that underground acid is usually quite pure. This finding contradicts popular belief, which holds that acid is frequently "cut" with strychnine, speed, or PCP.

Actually such contamination would rarely—if ever—occur. After all, it makes no economic sense to dilute acid with a drug that is *more* expensive to make—when acid itself, on a per-hit basis, is cheap to produce.

These drugs are just not potent enough to package in the forms in which acid commonly appears. An amount of speed, strychnine, or PCP strong enough for a consumer to feel simply won't fit into a microdot or onto a piece of blotter paper. Furthermore, the confirmed purity of "black market" acid is consistent with the philanthropic, idealistic motivations known to fuel the acid underground economy.

8

Acid Lingo

The acid experience may be fundamentally indescribable, but a lot of words and phrases have nonetheless been invented to describe it. The special vocabulary developed for the purpose of talking about acid and tripping is rich, creative, and colorful. The fact that a good portion of this lingo—from "turn on" to "trippy"—has worked its way into general usage indicates the enormity of the impact that acid and acid culture have had on society at large.

Acid Terminology

This entertaining series of terms used in the acid underground is adapted from a list collected by the DEA.

Acid head: Someone who takes LSD
Baby-sit: To guide someone through their first acid experience
Businessman's LSD: Dimethyltryptamine or "DMT," a short-acting psychedelic
Come home: To end an acid trip
Explorers club: A group of trippers
Frisco special: Heroin and acid

Ground control: The guide during a
psychedelic experience

Hits: Dosage units of acid, usually paper
squares

Lay the sheets: To apply acid to sheets of paper

Outer limits: Crack and acid

Satch: Papers, letters, cards, clothing, etc.,
saturated with acid   solution;
used to smuggle acid into prisons or
hospitals

Sheet rocking: Crack and LSD

Trails: A visual effect of acid that consists of
multiple images or trails that follow
moving objects

Travel agent: An acid dealer

Trips: Like "hits," dosage units of acid; usually
paper squares

Utopiates: Psychedelic drugs

Yen sleep: Restless, drowsy state after an acid
trip

Synonyms For Acid

Many words or phrases refer to the form in
which the acid is packaged or the image that appears on the blotter paper. The enormous length of
this list compiled by the DEA suggests that there
may be more synonyms for LSD than for any other
word in the English language!

*A, acid, animal, barrels, battery acid, beast, Big
D, black acid, black star, black sunshine, black tabs,
blotter, blotter acid, blotter cube, blue acid, blue
barrels, blue chairs, blue cheers, blue heaven, blue*

microdot, blue mist, blue moons, blue star, blue
vials, brown bombers, brown dots, California
sunshine, cap, chief, chocolate chips, cid, coffee,
conductor, contact lens, crackers, crystal tea, cubes,
cupcakes, d, deeda, domes, dots, double domes,
electric Kool-Aid, fields, flash, flat blues, ghost,
God's flesh, golden dragon, Goofy's, grape parfait,
green double domes, green single domes, green
wedge, gray shields, hats, Hawaiian sunshine,
hawk, haze, headlights, heavenly blue, instant Zen,
l, lason sa daga, LBJ, lens, lime acid, little smoke,
Logor, Lucy in the sky with diamonds, lysergide,
mellow yellow, Mickey's, microdot, mighty Quinn,
mind detergent, one way, optical illusions, orange
barrels, orange cubes, orange haze, orange micro,
orange wedges, Owsley, Owsley's acid, pane, paper
acid, peace, peace tablets, pearly gates, pellets, pink
blotters, pink Owsley, pink panther, pink robots,
pink wedge, pink witches, potato, pure love, purple
barrels, purple flats, purple haze, purple hearts,
purple ozoline, recycle, royal blues, Russian sickles,
sacrament, Sandoz, smears, snowmen, squirrel,
strawberries, strawberry fields, sugar, sugar cubes,
sugar lumps, sunshine, tabs, tail lights, ticket, trip,
25, vodka acid, wedding bells, wedges, white dust,
white lightning, white Owsley's, window glass,
windowpane, yellow, yellow dimples, yellow subma-
rine, yellow sunshine, Zen, Zig Zag man.

Psychedelic Expressions

Peter Stafford's *Psychedelics Encyclopedia* has a
list of words and phrases initially associated closely
with acid experience and culture that have found
their way into mainstream English popular usage.

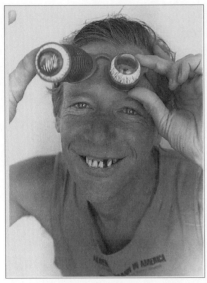

Peter Stafford

The list was compiled by Lester Grinspoon and James Bakalar, authors of *Psychedelics Reconsidered*. Here are some of the entries:

Turned on, straight, freak, freaked out, stoned, tripping, tripped out, spaced out, far out, flower power, ego trip, going with the flow, laying a trip on someone, mind-blowing, mind games, bringdown, centering, bum trip, karma, rapping, downer, flash, scene, vibes, great white light, doing your own thing, going through changes, uptight, getting into spaces, wiped out, where it's at.

9

Psychedelic Vines

 Morning Glory and Baby Hawaiian Woodrose are vines of the bindweed family which produce beautiful, brightly-colored blossoms. Their seeds contain high concentrations of lysergic acid amides, natural substances bearing a close resemblance in chemical structure to LSD. While the psychoactive effects of LSD and lysergic acid amides are very similar, LSD is fifty to one hundred times more potent than its natural chemical cousins.

More than five hundred species of the bindweed family have been identified around the world. The use of these plants by indigenous peoples for their psychoactive properties, however, has been documented only in the New World.

Sacred "Round Things" of the Aztecs

The Morning Glory vine is native to Central America and southern Mexico. Tribes native to these regions use the Morning Glory seed in rituals as an *entheogen*—a substance that generates inner experiences of God, gods, or divinity.

The Spanish Conquistadors conquered Mexico in 1521. Over the next century, a number of Spanish

writers described the use in religious ceremonies of
seeds called *ololiuqui*—meaning "round things"—by

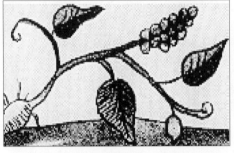

Snake Plant of the Aztecs

Aztecs and other
tribes. These seeds
came from a vine
that the natives
called *coaxihuitl*,
or "snake plant."
Native practice
sometimes com
bined the seeds of
the "snake plant"
with other entheogens, including mushrooms,
peyote, and Datura or "Jimson weed." The seeds
alone were particularly associated with the practice
of divination. In addition to entheogenic uses, natives have also employed Morning Glory seeds in
the treatment of gout and a malaria-like disease
called "aquatic fever."

From all of the descriptions penned by scribes
and explorers who followed after the Conquistadors
into the New World, it is clear that *ololiuqui* came
from a plant of the bindweed or Morning Glory
family. Most Spanish writers and documentarians,
however, didn't assign much importance to native
religious and medicinal practice. Botanical notes by
a physician named Hernandez which described the
veneration in which the natives held *ololiuqui* were
published in 1615. The publisher, however, all but
dismissed the observations of Hernandez with the
comment: "It matters little that this plant be here
described or that Spaniards be made acquainted
with it."

Due to such attitudes, knowledge of the Morning Glory seed's psychoactive powers was subsequently lost to all but a handful of Indian tribes for the next three hundred years.

Morning Glory Rediscovered

In 1897, *ololiuqui* was identified as the seed of Rivea corymbosa, the Mexican Morning Glory. This finding was definitively confirmed in 1939 by Richard Evans Schultes, a Harvard University ethnobotanis who has played an important role in advancing the world's knowledge of psychoactive plants. In 1955, Humphrey Osmond, the psychiatrist who coined the term "psychedelic,"

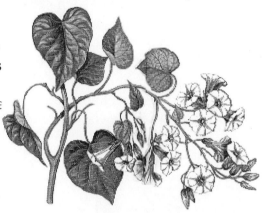

Rivea Cortmbosa, the Mexican Morning Glory

verified the psychoactivity of the seeds of the Mexican Morning Glory by ingesting them himself.

Chemical analysis of the seeds performed as a follow-up to Osmond's self-experimentation, however, failed to demonstrate the presence of any psychoactive substances. MK-ULTRA, the same secret CIA project that was experimenting with LSD as a weapon and mind-control agent, was interested in the seeds, but had similarly failed to identify their secret psychedelic ingredients.

Then, in 1959, Schultes sent a sample of seeds he had collected in Mexico to Albert Hofmann, the Swiss chemist who discovered LSD. Hofmann's analysis revealed that the seeds contained some of the same psychoactive alkaloids found in the rye mold—*ergot*—from which LSD had first been derived.

It seemed unlikely that chemicals previously found only in ergot would turn up in the morning glory—an organism of such radically different biology. For this reason and because earlier efforts had failed to find psychoactive components in the seeds, many scientists were skeptical of Hofmann's findings. Other chemists nonetheless confirmed his results, and the ergot alkaloids ergine, isoergine, chanoclavine, elymoclavine, and lysergol were identified as the psychoactive ingredients of the Mexican Morning Glory.

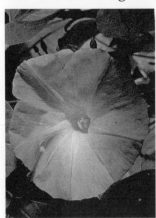

Ipomoea violecea

Sacramental use of another species of Morning Glory—*Ipomoea violacea*—by Zapotec Indians was reported around the same time that Hofmann analyzed the constituents of Rivea *corymbosa*. Zapotec ritual required that these seeds be ground up by a virgin when being prepared for use. In fact, the Zapotecs called the seed of Ipomoea violacea "the seed of the virgin." The seed of this morning glory species turned out to contain a roster of active ingredients almost identical to that of *ololiuqui*—but in much higher concentrations.

Over the next several years, word of these discoveries filtered into the psychedelic underground, and the practice of using Morning Glory seeds and extracts made from them to get high began to spread. Statements like "seed contained herein is for planting purposes only" began to appear on commercial packages containing Morning Glory seeds.

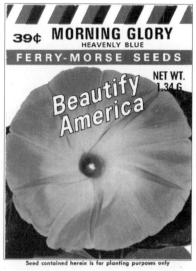

Seed contained herein is for planting purposes only

Morning glory seeds have been available in nurseries for years

Baby Hawaiian Woodrose

Seeds of another member of the bindweed family—the Baby Hawaiian Woodrose vine— have been discovered to contain much higher concentrations of lysergic acid amides than Morning Glory seeds. Baby Hawaiian Woodrose is a woody climbing vine with silvery foliage, purple flowers, and caramel-colored seed pods that flowers in August and

Baby Hawaiian Woodrose vine

early September. This bindweed is native to India, but is cultivated throughout the tropical regions of the world. It grows wild in the Hawaiian Islands, where it thrives in dry areas at lower elevations. Indigenous peoples of Hawaii are known to use the seed of the Baby Hawaiian Woodrose for entheogenic purposes.

A tantalizing hint left by a deceased master of meditation suggests that the Hawaiian Woodrose may have an ancient spiritual connection. The *Vedas*, Hindu religious texts more than a thousand years old, make awed references to an intoxicating plant concoction called *Soma*. The yogis and sages of old used this divine elixir to enhance their connection with God and assist them in their spiritual develop- ment. The use of Soma supposedly disappeared with the passage of the centuries, and the identity of the plant from which it came is therefore a mystery. Several scholarly theses and debates have been devoted to identifying the Soma plant, but no defini- tive conclusions have ever been reached.

In the early 1980s, a famous LSD researcher went to India and asked an elderly world-renowned guru of Yoga if he knew anything about the mysterious Soma. The spiritual teacher replied that he had been in contact with a obscure, remote sect of yogis who still practiced the entheogenic use of Soma, having secretly preserved the tradition for centuries. The swami said that the plant was a "creeper"—or vine—and promised that he would take the LSD researcher on a trek to see the plant for himself and meet the yogis who used it.

10

Tripping On Seeds

 The trips generated by Morning Glory and Baby Hawaiian Woodrose seeds are very similar to acid trips. With seeds, however, it takes one and a half to two hours after ingestion for psychedelic effects to set in, as opposed to an hour or less for acid. Seeds often cause side effects that are absent with acid, and seed trips usually have a tranquilizing quality not characteristic of acid.

Side Effects

Many trippers experience nausea, sometimes accompanied by vomiting—somewhat similar to the peyote experience—shortly after seeds are ingested. These side effects, however, generally disappear as the trip gets underway.

While some people feel enlivened after a seed trip, others experience a kind of hangover. Symptoms can include dizziness, lethargy, constipation, queasiness, and blurry eyesight. These after-effects usually dissipate by the end of the day after the trip.

Readers should be alerted that some of the active ingredients in Morning Glory and Baby Hawaiian Woodrose seeds can cause contractions of the uterus. This potential side effect presents a serious risk to pregnant women, who should not consume these seeds or extracts made from them under any circumstances.

According to Stafford in the *Psychedelics Encyclopedia*, excessive dosages of Morning Glory and Baby Hawaiian Woodrose have been associated with the appearance of a bluish color in the skin of the extremities. This phenomenon is consistent with loss of circulation, an effect which underlies the medical use of ergot alkaloids—as the active ingredients in the seeds are sometimes called—to prevent postpartum bleeding. Smart seed trippers avoid loss of circulation by approaching dosage judiciously. The determination of dosage is discussed in "Preparation and Use."

More "Mellow" Than Acid

Seed trips are often described as especially "relaxing" or "mellow" in comparison to the stimulating effects of LSD. Some trippers say that the seeds are in this aspect more akin to psychedelic mushrooms than acid.

Trippers often find that they can get to sleep much more quickly after a seed trip than after an acid trip. And while going to sleep during an acid trip is almost unheard of, some trippers have actually fallen asleep while still feeling strong psychedelic effects from seeds.

The relatively mellow character of seed trips may be due to the presence of a substance called *ergine*. Albert Hofmann investi gated this chemical in the 1940s

ergine

as part of his research into the chemistry of the ergot fungus, from which ergine takes its name. Ergine is the primary active ingredient in *ololiuqui*, the Mexican Morning Glory used as an entheogen by the Aztecs, and is present in the other psychedelic strains of Morning Glory as well as in Baby Hawaiian Woodrose. In addition to its psychedelic properties, ergine has pronounced sedative—in other words, tranquilizing—effects.

A Morning Glory Story

There are very few published accounts of seed trips. The following story involves a crop of Morning Glory seeds of historical significance—grown, harvested, and used for tripping by Timothy Leary and his companions on the grounds of the legendary Millbrook psychedelic retreat center in upstate New York.

More than a dozen years after the Millbrook experiment had disbanded, a well-known novelist indirectly connected to the Millbrook scene still possessed a large stash of these seeds. One summer Saturday, three of his young tripper friends—two women and a man—found out about this gold mine. They persuaded him to give them a generous portion of his stash, help them prepare the seeds for tripping, and remain on hand to guide their trip.

That evening the trio tripped with the guidance of their novelist friend. The two women experienced nausea—one of them vomited—but these side effects soon gave way to powerful, enjoyable trips.

But the young man—who had ingested the same quantity of seeds—still felt no effects at a time when his tripping partners were already very high. He remedied this situation by taking a second dose, almost as large as the first. In short order—and, by contrast, without any associated nausea—he blasted off on a very powerful psychedelic trip.

The nature of his experience, however, differed sharply from the relaxed, sedate quality usually ascribed to seed trips. In fact, he became almost uncontrollably stimulated. For several hours he darted constantly from room to room, conversation to conversation, and in and out of doors in such a cyclone of activity that his fellow trippers and his guide—who more than once during the course of the trip had to rescue him from zooming out into the street on foot—had trouble keeping track of him. Furthermore, he was hyped up not just *physically* but *sexually*. This normally shy, strictly heterosexual young man made sexual overtures not only to *both* of his female tripping companions, but to his male guide as well!

This tripper's overstimulation, however, in no way lessened the psychedelic qualities of his trip. At the peak of the trip he experienced himself to be God creating the universe out of the Void, using His own consciousness for building materials—a formative episode which led directly to study of Eastern spirituality and meditation.

But why did this tripper get so "speedy" when most people find seed trips so "mellow"? This little mystery highlights the unpredictable, sometimes downright contradictory nature of psychedelic experiences.

11
Cultivation

Morning Glories grow wild in many places and are cultivated in home gardens all around the United States. Baby Hawaiian Woodrose grows only in tropical and semi-tropical climates, making most of North America unsuitable for outdoor cultivation of this plant.

While commercially-obtained Morning Glory and Baby Hawaiian Woodrose seeds are often treated with fungicides and pesticides that make them inappropriate for human consumption, vines are grown from treated stock to yield seed harvests free from such contamination.

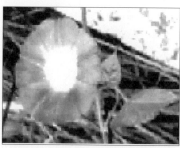

Morning Glory in bloom

Active Strains

Different varieties of Morning Glory produce seeds that vary widely in psychedelic potency. Strains with substantial psychoactive content include Flying Saucers, Heavenly Blue, Pearly Gates, Summer Skies, Wedding Bells, and Blue Star.

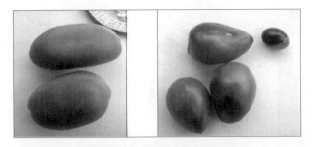

Seeds of the large Hawaiian Woodrose plant
contain much lower concentrations of lysergic acid
amides than the seeds of its close relative, the Baby
Hawaiian Woodrose (upper right).

Maximizing Psychoactive Potency

The combination of genetic factors, environmental conditions, and soil chemistry create as much as a sixteenfold variation in the psychoactive potency of seeds produced. Hormone treatment and attention to soil conditions and nutrients, however, go a long way toward maximizing the lysergic acid amide content of the seed harvest.

The same soil conditions, nutrients, and hormones that foster production of lysergic acid amides in Morning Glories are used to enhance the psychedelic content of Baby Hawaiian Woodrose seeds in regions—like Hawaii—that are sufficiently tropical for the successful cultivation of this plant.

Soil pH and Nutrients

The ideal soil pH, or soil acidity, for producing seeds of high potency is around 6.5. Soil pH test kits are sold at nurseries and gardening supply outlets, which also sell formulas for adjusting soil pH levels.

Soils high in nitrogen and phosphates and low in potassium produce seeds of high lysergic acid amide

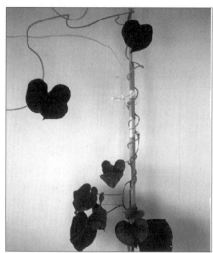

Baby Woodrose vine growing indoors

content. Ideal soil potassium content for this purpose is approximately 1.5 parts per 100 parts dry soil. Soil tests kits sold at nurseries and gardening supply outlets are used to check soil levels of nitrogen, phosphates, and potassium. Individual nutrients as well as nutrient formulas sold at these locations are used to adjust soil levels of these substances.

In order to keep soil potassium content low, cultivators use sodium nitrate instead of potassium nitrate as a nitrogen source, and use sodium acid phosphate—as opposed to potassium acid phosphate—as a phosphate source.

Hormones

Treatment with a hormone called gibberellic acid is used to maximize the lysergic acid amide content of the seed harvest. Gibberellic acid is obtained from chemical supply houses and is also found in formulas sold at nurseries.

Cultivators using formulas that contain gibberellic acid follow the instructions that come with the formula. Cultivators using pure gibberellic acid dissolve one gram in one liter of distilled water.

When the plants are still seedlings, they add a few drops of this solution to the soil around each plant before watering. They repeat this procedure every two weeks as the plant grows, using more solution each time until they are using about a half ounce of gibberellic acid per plant when the plants are fully grown.

Timing is an important aspect of treatment with gibberellic acid. Since this hormone delays the maturation of the plants and inhibits production of flowers and seeds, treatment is discontinued a few weeks before the plants are to flower.

A growth-inhibiting hormone called *alpha naphthalene acetic acid* is also used to increase the amount of lysergic acid amides present in the seeds.

Planting

Morning Glories are planted in the Spring when there is no longer any danger of frost. The cultivation process starts by soaking the seeds in water overnight. An alternative to soaking is to nick the coating of the seed with a sharp blade.

The seeds are planted about one-half inch deep and at least six inches apart in fine, loosely-packed, light-textured soil. As the vines grow, they are supported on trellises,

Harvesting

Baby Hawaiian Woodrose plants produce two crops of seeds every year. Morning Glory seeds are harvested in the Fall at the end of the growing season, when the concentration of lysergic acid amides is at its highest. Morning Glory seeds are ripe when they have become dark and hard.

12

Preparation and Use

Morning Glory and Baby Hawaiian Woodrose seeds are sold by stores and mail-order companies that offer seeds of decorative plants. Commercial seeds, however, are usually treated with fungicides or insecticides that make them dangerous for people to consume. Information about chemical additives is usually displayed on the package in which the seeds are sold.

Legal problems can result from the possession of ground-up seeds, which can be taken as evidence that the seeds are not being used for purely horticultural purposes and are intended for human consumption or chemical extraction.

Toxic Chemicals

Using commercial seeds for tripping is risky. People who do so wash them with soap and water, followed by a thorough water rinse, to remove the chemicals with which they have been treated. More cautious psychedelic seed enthusiasts, however, do not believe that such procedures provide adequate protection against toxic compounds and use only seeds that they have cultivated themselves or have been purchased from companies specializing in untreated seeds.

Potency and Dosage

Before ingesting the seeds, trippers determine an appropriate amount to consume. This decision is relatively easy if the tripper has previously used seeds from the same harvest or source and therefore knows how potent they are. Otherwise, dosage is a tricky issue because potency of both Morning Glory and Baby Hawaiian Woodrose seeds varies widely depending upon genetic and environmental factors.

Peter Stafford, author of *Psychedelics Encyclopedia*, equates the psychoactivity of one Morning Glory seed to that of one microgram or "mike" (millionth of a gram) of acid. By this standard, 65 Morning Glory seeds are required to produce a mild trip equivalent to that produced by the average 65-mike hit of acid, and 100 to 200 Morning Glory seeds are required for a strong psychedelic trip like that produced by 100 to 200 mikes of acid commonly taken in the 1960s.

Baby Hawaiian Woodrose seeds are much more potent than Morning Glory seeds. One Woodrose seed is roughly equivalent to 25 mikes of acid. In other words, two or three Woodrose seeds generate a mild trip like that produced by an average hit of acid, whereas four to eight seeds produce a more powerful trip equivalent to 100 to 200 mikes of acid.

When using an unfamiliar batch of seeds, most trippers prefer to err on the side of caution when it comes to dosage, selecting a quantity of seed that is more likely to be too little than too much. After they have already used seeds from a given batch, determining appropriate dosage becomes an easier matter.

Washing the Seeds

Even if the seeds haven't been treated with toxic chemicals, trippers still wash and rinse them before consumption in order to remove dirt and any other residues. Many prefer to use an all-natural soap product. After rinsing, the seeds are allowed to dry before further preparation.

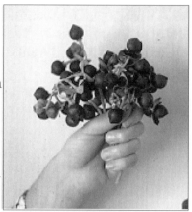

Baby Hawaiian Woodrose seed pods

How Seeds Are Prepared

Trippers thoroughly pulverize Morning Glory seeds before consuming them.They often use a common coffee grinder.

The ground seed is too gritty and unpleasant-tasting to be eaten dry, so trippers use a beverage to make a kind of morning glory seed shake. Most prefer beverages like milk or fruit juice that are more effective than water in masking the texture and taste. Trippers dump the dose of ground seed into a large tumbler of the beverage they have selected, stir the mixture vigorously, and then drink it down as fast as possible while it is still stirred up.

Aa an alternative to consuming the ground Morning Glory seed trippers soak them overnight in distilled water. They us distilled water because substances in tap water cause degradation of lysergic acid amides. The ground seed material is left in a cool, dark place while soaking to prevent decomposition of the amides by heat and light. They vigorously stir or shake the mixture several times while it is soaking.

The tripper pours the water off of the ground seed into a separate container—a process that chemists call decanting—or strains the liquid through a cheesecloth or other filter. Since lysergic acid amides are water-soluble, the run-off water contains active ingredients—a liquid infusion of the seed, a drink some people consume for psychedelic effect.

Since the infusion doesn't necessarily contain one hundred percent of the lysergic acid amides originally present in the seed, the trip it causes are not quite as strong as that which would occur from consuming an amount of ground seed equivalent to that from which the infusion was made. However, infusions cause less nausea and vomiting than consumption of ground seed.

How Seeds Are Consumed

Trippers pulverize Baby Hawaiian Woodrose seeds and which they put in a drink or use for an infusion just like Morning Glory seeds—with, of course, a much smaller number of seeds. Trippers experienced with Woodrose seeds, however, have discovered that such preparation is not necessary. Woodrose seeds do not have to be pulverized and swallowed in order to achieve psychedelic effects because their active ingredients are extracted by saliva and absorbed through the tissues of the mouth.

Trippers place the selected number of seeds in the mouth and then gently gnaw or lightly chew on them for a few minutes to break through the protective coating. Trippers then slide the seeds around the mouth like hard candy, hold them between cheek and gum like chewing tobacco, or slip them under the tongue like a sublingual medicine. After twenty minutes or more the seeds are removed from the mouth. Many trippers believe that this technique presents less chance of nausea than swallowing ground seeds.

Spitting while the seeds are still in the mouth or too soon after they have been removed may result in a loss of active ingredients. Drinking tap water or rinsing with it during this procedure may also be problematic because additives contained in tap water rapidly degrade lysergic acid amides into inactive substances.

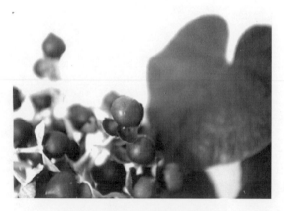

Baby Hawaiian Woodrose
pods and leaf

13

Psychedelic Seed Extracts

 Plant extracts are materials drawn out of plants by the wizardry of chemistry. Extracts feature high concentrations of specific desired substances that occur in much lower concentrations in the plants from which they are made. A very refined plant extract consists of a single chemical ingredient that has been carefully isolated and purified from the complex profusion of substances in the plant.

Many medicines are made by extraction from plants and other natural sources. Aspirin, for instance, comes from the bark of tree, and penicillin is extracted from a mold. Some alternative and homeopathic medicines are extracted from animal sources such as the glands of cows. With the advance of synthetic chemistry over the last half century, many medicines that first appeared as plant extracts are now produced from pure chemical "precursors"—or starting materials—instead of plant materials.

Psychedelic Extracts

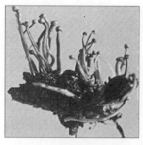

Magnified ergot

Extraction is the first stage of the process by which certain chemicals are synthesized in a laboratory. LSD, for instance, is made from *ergotamine tartrate,* a precursor extracted from a grain mold called ergot. Lysergic acid amides extracted from Morning Glory or Baby Hawaiian Woodrose seeds are an alternative starting material for LSD production.

Extractions of lysergic acid amides from seeds used for human consumption to produce psychedelic trips. This book documents the preparation and use of this kind of extract as opposed to the process of extraction performed as a stage of LSD production.

Side Effects

The trips that result from the use of seed extracts have the same general characteristics and potential side effects as trips that are produced by consuming the seeds themselves. Many trippers, however, believe that the incidence of side effects like nausea and vomiting is reduced by consuming extracts as opposed to the seeds.

RISK: The reader is alerted, however, that these extracts can cause uterine contractions just as readily as the seeds from which they are made and should therefore under no circumstances be consumed by pregnant women. Furthermore, the same constriction of circulation that has been connected to the use of excessive doses of seeds may also occur with the use of the extract.

Hazards of Extraction

Considerable skill, knowledge, care, and caution are required to safely extract lysergic acid amides from seeds. The solvent used and the vapor it emits are combustible, a hazard of special concern during the stage of the process when the solvent is being evaporated off. The solvent is also toxic—potentially lethal when ingested—and can be absorbed into the body by breathing its fumes. The lysergic acid amides being extracted can be absorbed through the skin in quantities sufficient to debilitate the chemist with their powerful psychedelic effects.

The solvent releases a tell-tale odor that can arouse suspicion and alert law enforcement. The reader should be reminded that both making and possessing lysergic acid amide extracts are against the law. Furthermore, since LSD can be made from lysergic acid amides, either of these crimes can be interpreted as evidence of an even more serious crime—the intent to manufacture LSD.

For all of these reasons, only qualified chemists who have special government licenses permitting them to work with lysergic acid amides should ever attempt the extraction process documented in this book, and they should do so only within the controlled conditions of a professional laboratory.

Quantity and Potency

The same process is used to extract active ingredients from both Morning Glory seeds and Baby Hawaiian Woodrose seeds. Woodrose seeds, however, are much more potent than Morning Glory seeds. An extraction from Woodrose seeds yields roughly three to six times the quantity of psychoactive chemicals produced by extracting a sample of Morning Glory seeds of the same weight.

The number of seeds that the chemist decides to use in the extraction depends to some extent on the number of doses desired. The extraction process, however, does not pull one hundred percent of the active ingredients out of the seed material. The number of seeds required to produce one dose of extract is therefore greater than the number required to produce a trip of the same strength when the whole seed is consumed. Just how much greater, however, isn't possible to determine with much accuracy in advance unless the alchemist has previously used the same extraction procedure on the same stock of seed and tested the potency of the result.

Even so, there is some margin of inconsistency in product potency each time the extraction is performed, especially with relatively elementary, low-tech procedures like the one documented in this book.

Since extraction is time-consuming and laborious, as well as hazardous, few alchemists undertake the process unless enough seeds are available to produce a generous number of doses. Several thousand Morning Glory seeds and a few hundred Woodrose seeds are the minimum numbers used to make an extraction process worthwhile.

Given that the profusion of variables involved severely limits the value of such estimates, one might hazard a guess that an efficiently executed extraction could produce a half-dozen mild trips from a hundred potent Baby Hawaiian Woodrose seeds or from two thousand potent Morning Glory seeds. The number of doses actually produced by an extraction, however, is determined only by laboratory analysis of the end product or by cautiously sampling it to see how strong it is.

Most alchemists keep a portion of seed stock in reserve for a second effort in case the first extraction gets botched.

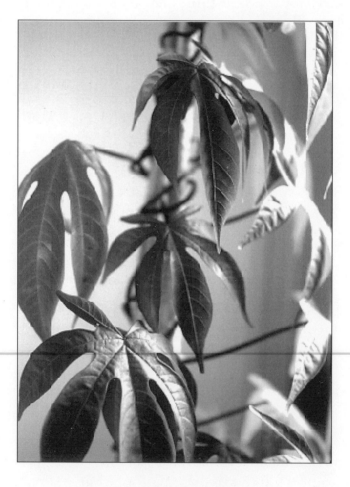

Large Hawaiian Woodrose vine

14

How Extracts Are Made

 Extracting lysergic acid amides from the protective environment of the seeds that contain them creates the risk of exposure to light and heat, which can cause rapid decomposition of the amides into inactive substances. For this reason, alchemists work quickly—but carefully—when extracting these sensitive psychedelic compounds from Morning Glory and Baby Hawaiian Woodrose seeds.

Seeds Are Washed

Before extraction begins, the alchemist washes the seeds with soap and cool distilled water, followed by a thorough rinse with cool distilled water, in order to remove dirt or other residues. The seeds are then allowed to dry out thoroughly.

Washing the seeds doesn't guarantee complete removal of the toxic insecticides and fungicides with which commercial seeds are sometimes treated. To prevent any traces of these poisons from finding their way into the final extract, most chemists use only untreated seeds.

Seeds Are Pulverized

The alchemist pulverizes the dried seeds in a flour mill, coffee grinder or food processor to produce a fine powder. Pulverizing Morning Glory seeds is relatively easy. Baby Hawaiian Woodrose seeds, which resemble hard little nuts, are more difficult to pulverize, so some chemists use a hammer to crack their hard casing before grinding them up.

Pet Ether Slurry

Then the alchemist places the pulverized seeds in a glass jar and pours in a solvent called *petroleum ether* is poured in. Petroleum ether, called "pet ether" for short, is poisonous and flammable. DANGER: Some varieties of petroleum ether boil at room temperature, releasing toxic and explosive fumes. This severe danger requires that the pet ether be stored in a freezer and poured only when ice-cold.

Generally, the alchemist uses about one milliliter (ml) of pet ether per seed. In the case of Woodrose seeds, which are larger than most varieties of Morning Glory seed and contain more active ingredients, up to two ml of pet ether is sometimes used.

After the pet ether is added, the alchemist seals the jar. The material inside is what chemists call a *slurry*, a very viscous mixture of soluble and insoluble substances in a solvent.

The chemist shakes the sealed slurry vigorously and then lets it sit for about twenty minutes, shaking it occasionally to maintain the material in a thoroughly mixed state.

Filtering

The alchemist pours the slurry through a funnel with filter paper in it. The funnel is made of glass because metals and plastics can react with pet ether, contaminating it with unwanted substances. A second glass jar placed underneath the funnel is used to collect the filtrate, the material that has passed through the filter.

The alchemist washes any material remaining in the first jar after pouring into the filter paper with additional pet ether.

The alchemist seals the jar in which the pet ether filtrate has been collected and refrigerated in order to save the pet ether, which is reusable.

The Filter Cake Is Dried

The alchemist collects the powdery solid left in the filter—called the *filter cake*— and leaves it out for the pet ether to evaporate off. The alchemist is always careful to dry the material thoroughly because toxic pet ether can find its way into the final extract.

DANGER: The pet ether fumes that are evaporating off during this stage of the procedure are both flammable and toxic. Because of these dangers, the chemist is careful to provide adequate ventilation.

The dried filter cake that remains after the solvent has evaporated off is the material from which the lysergic acid amides are extracted.

Alcohol Is Added

Extraction begins by adding high-proof alcohol to the thoroughly dried powder. Professional chemists use 100 percent reagent grade ethanol. Underground chemists sometimes use 150 proof rum or vodka or Ever Clear, an extremely high-proof alcoholic beverage which, due to its potency, is available only by mail order in some regions. Approximately 1 ml of alcohol is used for every Morning Glory or Woodrose seed that was pulverized for extraction. With lower proof alcohol, up to 1.5 ml per seed is used.

Extraction

The alcohol-filter cake mixture is allowed to sit for three days, during which time it is frequently and vigorously shaken. Between shakings, the alchemist stores the mixture in a cool, dark place to help prevent decomposition of the lysergic acid amides it contains.

The Extract Is Filtered

After three days have passed, the alchemist filters the mixture. He discards the filter cake and retains the liquid filtrate—the finished lysergic acid amide extract.

When held in sunlight or under an ultraviolet bulb, this psychedelic tincture radiates an aquamarine glow which indicates the presence of lysergic acid amides

How The Extract Is Used

The extract that has been produced has a very high alcohol content. RISK: Consuming too much can cause alcohol poisoning, which trippers use caution to avoid.

Since the potency of the extract is uncertain, a series of cautious experiments are usually undertaken to ascertain the appropriate dosage.

RISK: Excessive doses of lysergic acid amides may be associated with loss of circulation. Experienced trippers usually start by ingesting a very small amount—perhaps just enough tincture to cover the bottom of a shot glass with the thinnest possible layer. The liquid is held in the mouth for awhile before swallowing which permits absorption into the bloodstream of active ingredients through the tissues of the mouth.

If the quantity ingested in the first experiment proves to be insufficient, a second experiment is conducted a few days later using a slightly larger amount—and so on until a desirable dosage level has been determined.

To evaluate dosage accurately, two important factors are considered. First, it takes a few hours after ingestion for the full effects of lysergic acid amides to kick in. Second, people develop tolerance to LSD-type substances very quickly, so at least a few days must elapse between doses if the potency of the extract is to be assessed with any real precision.

Storage

Decomposition of the amides is minimized by refrigerating the extract when it is not being used and by keeping it in an opaque or darkly-tinted jar.

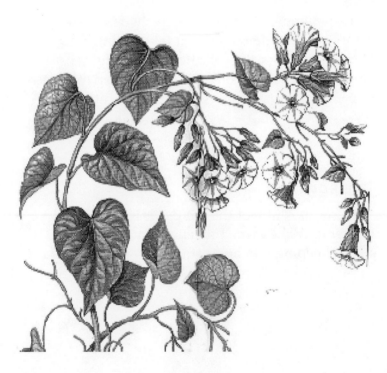

Rivea Cory

15

Acid, Seeds, and the Law

 Possession, sale, and manufacture of LSD, as well as lysergic acid amides—the psychedelic substances contained in Morning Glory and Baby Hawaiian Woodrose seeds—are illegal in the United States under the Federal Controlled Substances Act. Serious legal restrictions have also been placed on these substances in many other nations of the world.

The Controlled Substances Act

Acid was banned in the United States in 1967. Like all other extant Federal drug laws, however, the laws prohibiting LSD were superseded in 1970 by the Federal Controlled Substances Act. The purpose of this Act was to replace the inconsistent, fragmentary, and dated drug laws that had accumulated over the years with a systematic, unified, and comprehensive body of national legislation on the subject.

Schedules

The Federal Controlled Substances Act groups all controlled substances into five legal categories or "schedules," which are assigned the Roman numerals I through V. Drugs subject to the most severe legal restrictions are placed in Schedule I. Successively decreasing levels of legal restriction are associated with Schedules II through V. Drugs are grouped into one of the five categories according their abuse potential and the presence or absence of medical uses accepted within the United States.

LSD

The Controlled Substances Act assigns LSD to Schedule I. The law considers substances in this category to have high abuse potential and no accepted medical uses. Schedule I substances are also considered to be unsafe even when used under medical supervision. The manufacture, distribution, possession, import, and export of Schedule I drugs are felonies associated with the severest penalties to which drug crimes are subject.

Marijuana—despite its many medical applications—appears in Schedule I, as does heroin. Several psychedelics besides LSD are also classified in Schedule I, including peyote—a cactus sacred to several native American tribes for its visionary properties—and mescaline, peyote's psychoactive ingredient.

Carrier Weight

A particularly controversial aspect of LSD law has been the issue of "carrier weight." In many acid cases, the weight of the blotter paper, liquid, or other material that contains the acid—called the "carrier"—has been included with the weight of the acid itself which vastly increases the severity of the sentence handed down under mandatory sentencing laws, which base punishment on weight of the drug involved. The inclusion of carrier weight results in far greater sentences for LSD than for equivalent numbers of doses of other Schedule I substances—for instance, heroin—for which no carrier is required.

The practice of accounting for carrier weight in acid cases has condemned many people to more than twenty years in Federal prison for possession of only a few hundred hits—with no option of parole because of the mandatory minimums required for drug case sentencing. The inequity of this situation is highlighted by the fact that people convicted of murder are often placed on parole after only seven years.

Lysergic Acid Amides

The Federal Controlled substances Act assigns the lysergic acid amides found in Morning Glory and Baby Hawaiian Woodrose seeds to Schedule III, a category that also includes anabolic steroids. Substances in Schedule III are considered to have lower abuse potential than those in schedules I and II. These drugs have medical uses that are accepted within the United States. A Schedule III lysergic acid derivative called *methysergide*, for instance, is widely used for migraine headaches—in doses far too mild to cause psychedelic effects. It is illegal to possess Schedule III substances without a prescription or special government license.

Lysergic acid amides are sometimes used as starting materials in the production of LSD. Possession of these substances can therefore be used in court as evidence of intent to manufacture LSD—a very serious crime. Anyone who performs extraction of lysergic acid amides from seeds—including the procedure described in this book—therefore risks getting in serious legal trouble unless he or she possesses a license to work with these substances.

Morning Glory and Baby Hawaiian Woodrose Seeds

Because it is illegal to possess lysergic acid amides, it can also be illegal to possess the plants that contain them. The authorities, however, widely permit the possession of Morning Glory and Baby Hawaiian Woodrose plants and seeds for decorative horticultural purposes. Morning Glory seeds, for instance, are commonly—and legally—available from commercial seed companies, and Morning Glory plants are grown in gardens all over the country.

Intent

Legal and illegal possession of these plants and seeds are distinguished by law according to the issue of intent. It is a crime, for instance, to possess these plants with intent to ingest them—or extractions made from them—for their psychedelic effects. It is also a crime to possess these plants with intent to extract their ingredients for the production of LSD.

Intent is determined by available evidence. The possession of ground-up seeds, for example, can be taken as evidence of illegal intent because such material is used for human ingestion or chemical extraction but not for horticulture. The possession of solvents and other chemicals or hardware used in extraction or LSD production can also be taken as evidence that seeds are intended for illegal use.

Chemicals Used In Manufacture

Federal law also prohibits possession of chemicals used in illicit manufacture of controlled substances. These chemicals include starting materials or "precursors"—in the case of LSD, lysergic acid amides and ergotamine tartrate. Also included are compounds used in chemical reactions, known in legal terminology as "essential substances." Solvents can also be considered illegal if used or intended for use in the production of controlled substances.

Penalties and Sentences

The Federal Controlled Substances Act provides sentencing guidelines that judges are required to follow. Determining the sentence mandated for a given drug crime can require complex calculation. Factors that figure in the severity of the sentence include the quantity in terms of weight of controlled substance involved, the Schedule to which that substance belongs, whether or not weapons were seized, and the prior convictions—if any—of the person being sentenced. While judges have almost no latitude under mandatory sentencing, sentences can be decreased when the testimony of a convicted person is used to convict others.

Keeping Up With The Law

The interpretation and application of drug laws—like all other laws—change over time according to precedents established by specific court cases. Courts may also declare certain laws, or aspects of them, to be unconstitutional. Certainty about the current status of any law therefore requires keeping up with relevant court decisions.

An excellent source of information about laws and sentences applying to LSD, lysergic acid amides is *Controlled Substances: Chemical and Legal Guide to the Federal Drug Laws* by Alexander T. Shulgin. *Marijuana Law* by Richard Glen Boire contains a great deal of helpful information about drug law in general.